The Laws Of Gravity

Chronic Dieter's Edition

ROBIN ASHLEY LONG, C.A., M.ED.

Order this book online at www.trafford.com or www.Pro-ActiveCounselling.com
or email orders@trafford.com

Most Trafford titles are also available at major online book retailers.

Note for Librarians: A cataloguing record for this book is available from Library
and Archives Canada at www.collectionscanada.ca/amicus/index-e.html

Printed in Victoria, BC, Canada.

ISBN: 978-1-4269-1511-6

*Our mission is to efficiently provide the world's finest, most comprehensive book publishing
service, enabling every author to experience success. To find out how to publish your book, your
way, and have it available worldwide, visit us online at www.trafford.com*

Trafford rev. 12/21/2009

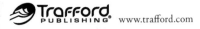

www.trafford.com

North America & international
toll-free: 1 888 232 4444 (USA & Canada)
phone: 250 383 6864 ♦ fax: 812 355 4082

A NOTE FROM THE AUTHOR

"Unfortunately, eating disruptions cause us to feel bad about who we are and separate us from our natural (pre-disrupted) state. Being disconnected from our internal emotional state causes us to put excess pressure on our external physical state. Eventually, we begin to identify solely with our external bodies and confuse this with our self-worth. To make matters worse, we are living in an appearance and weight obsessed society. Since our eating affects how we look, we are judged by our eating behaviours. Thus, in society's eye, we actually become our eating disturbance! We are graded on this physical form that does not represent who we would be in our natural state. The truth is that we are not our eating disturbance. How we eat is not the essence of who we are, but simply the behaviours that we engage in. We need to wake up and remind ourselves of this fact. We are born knowing, but somewhere along the way, we forget and submit to a more deprecating self-concept which causes us unnecessary pain and suffering. We need to become re-aligned with our natural selves and learn to live in a more natural manner, returning to our natural state."

- Excerpt, *The Laws Of Gravity*

"This book is devoted to enriching the quality of your days and your lives, resulting in improved physical and mental well-being, allowing you to create a better relationship with yourself and have a greater level of self-love, honour and respect."

I invite you to use these laws to assist you in creating your own synergistic path and I genuinely wish you the best of luck on your journey!

- Robin Ashley Long

FOREWORD

A fresh new perspective…..it is time for change.

It will take more than the right mix of foods to stop the harsh voices from within. It will require more than an exercise routine to eliminate punitive thoughts and destructive behaviours.

The Laws of Gravity offers a realistic alternative to quick fix dieting and weight loss solutions that rarely have a lasting effect. These *Laws* can actually change the way you relate to food and yourself. If you are ready to accept that no diet is the answer or the cure for your self-image issues and discontent, then you are ready for *The Laws of Gravity.*

This book provides the essential knowledge that individuals require to guard themselves against the magical illusions of dieting. It presents a fresh new perspective on some very basic, fundamental information about our eating rituals and relationships. You will learn a new script, a new way of thinking, living and being that can transform the defiant parts of you that are resistant to change.

Exceptionally well documented and explained, these *Laws* will prevent individuals from suffering unnecessarily. If properly utilized and put into practice, the potential for change is inevitable. There is a difference between knowing what to do and actually doing it. This book provides sufficient knowledge to understand the changes that are necessary as well as a road map that explains how to actualize these *Laws* and ultimately make them a natural part of your every day existence. It is through experiencing these simple but profound truths presented in this book, that people will come to benefit from *The Laws of Gravity.*

Robin is clearly dedicated to providing others with the tools that they need to move ahead and assisting them on their journey to a happier and healthier self, inside and out.

Dr. Stephanie Bot, C. Psych., Psychoanalyst

Table of Contents

The Laws Of Gravity - Chronic Dieter's Edition

A Global Phenomenon

On a global level, we have developed a self-destructive relationship with food, with one third of the world's population starving through famine and the rest of us, through self-inflicted deprivation. Globally, we have become obsessed with how we look and how we eat. By compulsively focusing on food, we are creating a state of psychological scarcity, where we constantly think we have too little and need too much. As such, our experiences around food are not satisfying and we are left psychologically hungry, regardless of how much we actually take in. We need to transform this process and create a more positive psychological state of abundance and availability so that we experience physical and psychological contentment and satiation. Ultimately, we must change the relationship that we have with food, our bodies and ourselves.

Food is a form of energy that we use to fuel our bodies and also a uniquely powerful stimulus of reward and punishment. Psychologically, we are feeding ourselves negative energy by swallowing our food with negative thoughts. We need to fuel our bodies with positive thoughts and positive energy in order to meet life's challenges with strength and optimism, instead of making eating a challenge in and of itself. There needs to be a shift in the way we feed our bodies and our minds, from negative to positive, from critical to accepting, from self-destructive to synergistic and from self-deprecating to self-respecting. We need to change the direction of our energy so that we can move one step forward, one step upward, one step at a time.

To redirect and change our path, we must re-align ourselves with our natural, pre-disrupted state, the way we would have been had our relationship with food never been disturbed. It is not the external behaviours that we need to focus on to create this shift, but our internal experiences that must change for us to permanently alter our relationship with food. We don't need to re-shape our bodies, we need to re-shape our minds and allow our bodies to follow.

To do this, we must ACKNOWLEDGE the process that we are engaging in and bring our actions into conscious awareness. We need to ACCEPT all of our past actions which have led us to our present state of being. We need to ALLOW our emotions to surface so that we can re-ALIGN with our true or Natural State and ARISE to a higher level of being. While it will take a concerted effort to change our conscious thinking at first, when fuelled by internal positive thoughts and experiences, rising above and spiraling upward will ultimately be effortless.

This is not a diet or weight loss book. The aim is not to deny or avoid hunger, but to clarify our experiences of it so that we can respond in as efficient a manner as possible. The purpose of this book is to assist us in enhancing our relationship with food. If we amend our goal of dieting into "transforming and enhancing the relationship that we have with ourselves", we can create a positive feedback system that is guaranteed to bring us success. This book is devoted to enriching the quality of our days and our lives, resulting in improved physical and mental well-being, allowing us to create a better relationship with ourselves and to have a greater level of self-love, honour and respect.

The Path To A More Satisfying Relationship With Food

PHASE I: ACKNOWLEDGEMENT
In this first phase, we need to understand our eating behaviours and bring the process into conscious awareness. We need to become aware of how our actions perpetuate themselves. Acknowledgement is the first step in our recovery. In this section we will realize that we can live in alignment with who we naturally are and live in harmony with our appetites, our bodies and ourselves.

PHASE II: SELF-ACCEPTANCE
The only way that we can develop a better relationship with food and begin an upward spiral of experiences surrounding eating is to change our internal psychological state. The difference between "spiraling up" and "spiraling down" is the presence or absence of positive thoughts which can only be achieved through self-acceptance. In this section we will see that the promise we make to "not abandon ourselves" is the most important commitment we can make.

PHASE III: ALLOW
Once we create a purely positive psychological state around eating, we will be able to stop the conscious mind from focusing on food. In the absence of this conscious distraction, the feelings that we have buried will be ALLOWED to surface. In this section we will see that allowing ourselves to feel is the most courageous act we can engage in.

CONCLUSION:
Once we RE-ALIGN ourselves with our natural appetite and deal directly with our emotions, we can arise to a more satisfying way of being.

Are You A Cycle – Path?

1. Do you experience an internal struggle with food?

2. Do you think about your meals after you have eaten?

3. Do you feel uneasy when you are not on a diet?

4. Do you put dieting rules ahead of your own?

5. Do you second guess your food choices?

6. Do you regret your food choices after you have eaten?

7. Do you think about food often?

8. Do you wish you could stop thinking about food?

9. Do you have difficulty figuring out when you are hungry?

10. Do you have difficult determining when you are full?

11. Do you over-eat?

12. If you over-eat do you continue to think about food?

13. Do you restrict or under-eat?

14. If you restrict or under-eat, do you continue to think about food?

15. Do you have difficulty being satiated after you have eaten?

16. When you are satiated, do you continue to think about food?

17. Do you feel guilty after you have eaten?

18. Do you judge yourself based on what you have eaten?

19. Do you feel tired often?

20. Is getting enough sleep an issue for you?

21. Is getting enough water an issue for you?

22. Do you have trouble experiencing emotions in the moment?

23. Are your emotional experiences confusing or unsatisfying?

24. Do you have difficulty accepting your body?

25. Do you put a great deal of effort into weight loss or maintenance?

26. Do you wish it was easier to maintain your weight?

27. Do you wish you had more control over your relationship with food?

28. Do you wish you had a different relationship with food?

29. Do you wish you had a different relationship with your body?

30. Do you wish you had a different relationship with yourself?

If you have answered yes to more than five of these questions, you are likely to unnecessarily suffer through some form of NEGATIVE CYCLING with respect to your relationship with food. You will be able to benefit from altering your experiences and obtain some relief from the detrimental thinking that has been disrupting your internal state.

Definitions

Pure Essence Eating is achieved when we offer our body what it needs when it needs it, when we respond accurately to physical or Chemical Hunger.

Body Maintenance System encompasses the entire spectrum of activities that affect our body, our body image, our weight, our metabolism and our self-perception.

Body Harmony is achieved when there is an alignment between the level of effort we put into Body Maintenance and the satisfaction that we obtain. As this system becomes more balanced and easier to maintain, we are able to engage in a more natural way of living and being.

Chemical Hunger: True physical hunger with an actual physiological cause. When properly responded to by food, the experience of hunger subsides and satiation is achieved.

Phantom Hunger: Psychological hunger; the experience of hunger without a physiological cause. Anything that causes us to think we are hungry for reasons other than physical need. When responded to by food, phantom hunger does not subside.

Diet: An external set of rules that dictate how and when we should eat. These rules override our internal appetite and alter the way that we respond to physical or Chemical Hunger.

Natural State: The relationship that we would have with food, our metabolisms, our bodies and ourselves had our eating patterns never been disrupted. We are in our Natural State when we are in alignment with our appetite and when we offer ourselves unconditional acceptance; not expecting ourselves to be anywhere else on our journey than where we are at this moment.

Synergy: To expand or make more. Synergy is created when things work together to produce an outcome that is of more value than the sum of the individual parts. Synergy is experienced through positive cycling.

De-synergize: To reduce or make less. This is the opposite of synergy. It represents our descent from grace (our Natural State) and the negative cycling that we experience when we enter into a lifestyle that is dictated by dieting.

Surface Emotions: Experiences that create drama and mask how we are really feeling.

True Emotions: Underlying essential emotions that tell us how we are really feeling.

NOTE: This book is not meant to discredit any one particular diet or negate any success that individuals have found with an eating regime. While it may be possible for some people to find a system that allows them to more easily respond to physical or Chemical Hunger, for many, this same system will lead to feelings of deprivation. The discerning factor is whether it enhances or inhibits our ability to identify and respond to our appetite and whether it prevents or assists us in developing a positive and healthy relationship with food. Please don't confuse healthy eating principles with an external set of rules that prevent an individual from responding to hunger. Know that it may be difficult to distinguish between Chemical and Phantom Hunger and that this may change through the duration of our healing journey.

The Laws Of Gravity

For those of us affected by struggles with dieting, our personal relationship with ourselves and our self-concept is dictated by our relationship with food and our bodies. Our relationship with food and our bodies is dictated by our relationship with ourselves and our self-concept. And the cycle repeats itself. We can call this, the original "spin"......the origins of which create the negative spinning that we, as dieters can experience, which causes our lives to spin out of control.

The Original "Spin" (Sin)

> Our personal relationship with ourselves and our self-concept is dictated by our relationship with food and our bodies.

> Our relationship with food and our bodies is dictated by our relationship with ourselves and our self-concept. And the cycle repeats itself...

These fundamental *Laws of Gravity* are whole truths that must be brought into our conscious awareness in order to help us understand our relationship with food, our bodies and ourselves. This will help us shift from a detrimental eating cycle to a more beneficial one. Having a series of pleasant experiences surrounding food will enable us to follow a more positive path. We can use these *Laws of Gravity* to give us the foundation and the ability to rise above, instead of allowing them to 'weigh' us down.

These laws do not change over time but are enduring forces of nature. We can`t use them until we "are fixed" and then ignore and discard them. They are always relevant, regardless of where we are in our journey. They do not represent new or ground-breaking information. They simply remind us of what we already know but have forgotten because of the distracting nature of our eating disturbances. It is in our best interest to find a way to understand, embrace, and work collaboratively with them so that we can support ourselves throughout our journey.

NOTE: The term "we" instead of "you" has been used throughout this book to signify inclusion and to reinforce the fact that the Laws of Gravity apply to all of us.

Phase One: Acknowledgement

1. **To optimize our relationship with food, we need to give our body what it needs when it needs it. (Pure Essence Eating)**

To strengthen and build the most beneficial relationship with food possible, we need to give our body what it needs when it needs it, without judgment and with full acceptance of our responses to hunger. This is known as Pure Essence Eating. Any gap that exists between our natural appetite and Pure Essence Eating will cause a disruption in the system and impair our ability to effectively nourish our bodies and achieve optimal Body Harmony, ultimately making weight maintenance more difficult. Understanding that we don't need to struggle to be who we are naturally, and that we can live in alignment with our appetite is a powerful realization.

GOAL: The goal of our eating system is to accurately experience, interpret and respond to our natural appetite.

BOTTOM LINE: By responding accurately to our appetite, we will optimize our relationship with food.

NOTE: The "Bottom Line" assists us in achieving our "Goal" and the cycle repeats itself.

2.   The nature of dieting causes the need for dieting.

Dieting separates us from our natural appetite and forces us to deny or manipulate our experiences of hunger. Dieters, more than any other group, listen to externally derived rules to determine what and when they need to eat. It is the willingness to allow dieting restrictions to override our appetite that is detrimental to our development. When we abide by dieting rules, we do not develop the skills necessary to interpret hunger and are therefore unable to accurately read, respond to and satiate our hunger. We then begin to question and second guess the hunger messages that we receive, which increases our dependency on the diet. Following a diet and ignoring our true appetite, ultimately causes the need to rely on external rules to guide our eating behaviours.

NEGATIVE CYCLE	POSITIVE CYCLE
Diets are an externally derived system of eating rules.	The appetite is an internally derived system of eating rules.
Enforcing an external eating system decreases our ability to interpret hunger.	Relying on an internal eating system increases our ability to interpret hunger.
Impairing our ability to interpret hunger prevents us from trusting our appetite and relying on ourselves.	Enhancing our ability to interpret hunger allows us to trust our appetite and rely on ourselves.
Our inability to rely on ourselves causes the need to depend on external rules and the cycle repeats itself.	Our ability to rely on ourselves decreases the need to depend on external rules and the cycle repeats itself.

GOAL: To rely on our internal appetite to tell us what and when we need to eat.

BOTTOM LINE: The only way to improve our ability to read our appetite is to rely on it over externally derived rules.

3. Ruminating about food increases our experience of hunger.

As dieters, we spend an excessive amount of time thinking about what we have eaten and what we will eat, regardless of whether or not we are in fact hungry. Our minds are, more often than not, preoccupied by thoughts of food. Ruminating about food stimulates the appetite and causes the experience of hunger whether or not our bodies actually need nourishment, making the whole hunger management process and Body Maintenance System more difficult.

There are two types of hunger, physical or Chemical Hunger and psychological or Phantom Hunger. Chemical Hunger is the body's way of letting us know what and when we need to eat. Responding to Chemical Hunger will enable us to maximize our metabolism, have pleasurable eating experiences and send positive messages to the self. Failing to respond to Chemical Hunger causes us to ruminate about food until the craving is satisfied. The greater the delay in responding to Chemical Hunger, the more hunger will be experienced. As dieters, we have become separated from our natural appetite and have lost or failed to develop the ability to accurately read and respond to Chemical Hunger. Because we often do not give our bodies what they need, we are likely to experience Chemical Hunger more often than necessary.

Any messages that have no physiological origin, yet are interpreted by the brain as hunger, are psychological or Phantom Hunger. Responding to psychological or Phantom Hunger by eating cannot be satisfying because we aren't actually hungry. If we weren't hungry before we ate it, we won't be satisfied after we have eaten it. This explains why we can eat food without becoming satiated and why we can continue to think about food after we have eaten. It is Phantom Hunger that ultimately leads us to feeling deprived, regardless of how much we have consumed.

Simply put, if we constantly experience hunger and think about eating food, we must restrict our cravings and are therefore left feeling deprived in some manner. If we occasionally experience hunger and think about eating food, we may respond to our wishes and are therefore left feeling satisfied.

NEGATIVE CYCLE	POSITIVE CYCLE
The more we think about food the more the appetite is stimulated.	The less we think about food, the less the appetite is stimulated.
The more the appetite is stimulated, the more hunger we will experience.	The less the appetite is stimulated, the less hunger we will experience.
Continuously thinking about food causes us to live in a state of perceived deprivation where we constantly experience hunger regardless of how much we are actually feeding ourselves.	Not thinking about food enables us to live primarily in a state of **satiation, where we** experience hunger only when we truly physically require nourishment..
Responding to Phantom Hunger does not eliminate it or stop us from thinking about food. We continue to ruminate and the cycle repeats itself.	Responding to Chemical Hunger eliminates it and stops us from thinking about food and the cycle repeats itself.

GOAL: To clarify our experience of hunger.

BOTTOM LINE: The less time we spend thinking, fretting, planning, strategizing and scheming about food, the clearer our experiences of hunger will be.

4. Each and every time we respond to hunger we send a message to the self. Each message either strengthens or weakens our relationship with our appetite.

We always respond to hunger whether we feed it or not. We may eat or refuse to eat, but all actions (or non-actions) are a psychological response to hunger. Our goal is to be fully aware about what our responses are and to be careful about the messages that we send ourselves. To do this we need to bring these thoughts into conscious awareness.

The first response to hunger is a thought, not an action. Pure Essence Eating thrives in an environment of positive thinking and is fueled by encouraging thoughts. What we do is of much less importance than our psychological state while we are doing it. If our thoughts are restrictive and judgmental, we will head into a negative cycle by feeling deprived and constantly ruminating about food. If our thoughts are of abundance and acceptance, we can create pleasurable experiences surrounding food and eating and follow a path that requires a lot less effort (the path of least resistance). This is regardless of how much or how little we have consumed.

NEGATIVE CYCLE (Phantom Hunger is enhanced by a negative reinforcement system.)	POSITIVE CYCLE (Chemical hunger is enhanced by positive reinforcement system.)
Failing to read and respond accurately to hunger on a timely basis sends a negative message to the self.	Accurately interpreting and responding to hunger on a timely basis sends a positive message to the self.
Negative messages separate us from our appetite and decrease the trust we have in our ability to feed ourselves.	Positive messages reinforce our connection to our appetites and increase the trust we have in our ability to feed ourselves.
The less trust we have in our ability to feed ourselves, the less likely we will be to listen to our appetites.	The more faith we have in our ability to feed ourselves, the more likely we will be to listen to our appetites.
The less we listen to our appetites, the less appetite clarity we will have and the more difficult it will be to accurately respond to it. And the cycle repeats itself.	The more we listen to our appetites, the more appetite clarity we will have and the easier it will be to accurately respond to it. And the cycle repeats itself.

GOAL: To strengthen our relationship with our appetite by offering ourselves positive thoughts surrounding our responses to hunger.

BOTTOM LINE: The more we positively reinforce our actions by sending positive messages to ourselves, the more likely we will be to trust our appetite and strengthen our connection to it.

5. Under-eating leads to over-eating and over-eating
    leads to under-eating.

More accurately phrased, physical and/or psychological under or
over-eating, leads to physical and/or psychological under or over-
eating.

Under and over-eating are both unnatural physical responses to
physical hunger and are detrimental to both the psyche and the
metabolism. The same psychological process initiates an "inaccurate
response" to hunger. Whether the path of "more" or "less" is chosen is
irrelevant. The end result is the same, a separation from the self.

As dieters, more than any other group of individuals, we fail to
respond to hunger signals and instead, offer ourselves what we
think we 'should' eat. Playing games with our hunger and ultimately
eating what we don't want is not satisfying. **"Fake food causes
frustration, not satiation." "Calories that don't
count, don't leave us content."** If we restrict when we are
hungry, we will make up for it by eating food that we don't want at
times when we don't need it, because **denial creates desire**.
This in turn causes guilt and the desire to restrict. As dieters, we
therefore tend to both over and under- eat.

To complicate matters, once separated from our appetite, the actual
concepts of too much and too little become skewed. This phenomenon
starts to play itself out on a psychological level which inhibits our
ability to read our appetite accurately. Feelings of deprivation lead
to rebellion and over-eating. Thoughts of over-indulgence lead to
feelings of guilt and the desire to restrict. Once again, the result is
the same, a further separation from the appetite and from the self.

5a) Denial Creates Desire – with restrictions, come hunger.

(Under-Eating Cycle)

NEGATIVE CYCLE	POSITIVE CYCLE
Real and/or perceived under-eating causes real and/or perceived hunger.	Giving our bodies what they need when they need it (Pure Essence Eating) allows us to be physically satiated.
The more hunger we experience, the more likely we will be to over-eat.	The more satiated we are, the less likely we are to experience hunger and the less likely we are to over-eat.
The more we over-eat, the more likely we will feel the need to restrict and to under-eat. And the cycle repeats itself.	The less we over-eat, the less we will feel we need to restrict and more likely we will be to respond to hunger. And the cycle repeats itself.

5b) Feast Leads to Famine – with indulgence, comes guilt.

(Over-Eating Cycle)

NEGATIVE CYCLE	POSITIVE CYCLE
Real and/or perceived over-eating causes guilt and the desire to restrict intake in the future.	Giving our bodies what they need when they need it (Pure Essence Eating) allows us to be physically satiated.
Restricting or the threat of future restrictions causes ruminations about food and increases hunger.	The more satiated we are, the less likely we are to experience hunger and the less likely we are to over-eat.
The more hunger we experience, the more likely we will be to over-eat. And the cycle repeats itself.	The less we over-eat, the less we will feel we need to restrict and more likely we will be to respond to hunger. And the cycle repeats itself.

With repetition, comes realization: Please note the similarity of the charts for Laws 5, 6 and 7.

GOAL: To accurately read and respond to hunger.

THE BOTTOM LINE: The more we focus on our experiences of hunger in the present moment, the better we will be able to accurately respond to it.

6. **In the absence of restricted eating, "want" and "need" become one. Under the influence of restricted eating, "want" takes over and "needs" are ignored.**

As dieters, we feel that we will never be able to eat what we want. We feel guilty and ashamed for wanting too much, as though it is in some way unnatural or unhealthy. However, it is the limitations that we place on ourselves that inflate our desire in the first place. In the absence of such restrictions, our "wants" and our "needs" become one. At some point, the rules that we believe keep us "diet safe" turn on us and lead us to both over and under-eat, causing the whole Body Maintenance System to become far too difficult.

For many of us, the mere suggestion of food restrictions sends us into a Phantom Hunger frenzy and creates an intense desire for the very foods that we try to restrict. This stems from an underlying fear that we will not respond to Chemical Hunger and will not get our physical needs met. The mind rejects the idea of external restrictions, even if they are only perceived restrictions with little or no physical validity.

Simply put, when we fear that food is unavailable to us, we are more likely to crave it, whether we physically need it or not. On the flip side, when we know that food is available to us, we are more likely to eat it when we are hungry for it. Feeding true Chemical Hunger is always more satisfying that feeding Phantom Hunger because food tastes best and is most satiating when our body needs it.

NEGATIVE CYCLE	POSITIVE CYCLE
Restricting or the threat of future restrictions causes fear, anxiety, ruminations about food and increases hunger.	In the absence of restrictions, we are able to respond accurately to hunger and give our body what it needs to become satiated.
The more hunger we experience, the more likely we will be to over-eat or to restrict. And the cycle repeats itself. (Loop #1)	The more satiated we are, the less likely we are to think about food and the less hunger we will experience.

The more we over-eat, the more guilt we will experience and the more likely we will be to feel the need to restrict in the future. And the cycle repeats itself. (Loop #2)	The less hunger we experience, the less we will feel we need to restrict and more likely we will be to respond accurately to hunger. And the cycle repeats itself.

GOAL: To align hunger with desire.

BOTTOM LINE: Restrictions inflate desire, causing the need to restrict.

7. **Guilt ultimately increases hunger and detrimentally affects our relationship with food, our bodies and ourselves.**

Guilt begets guilt.

Guilt deserves some extra attention due to the detrimental affect it has on the psyche and on our eating behaviours. Guilt is one of the leading causes of Phantom Hunger and one of the main sources of negative messages to the self. These messages start the negative spiraling, creating a de-synergistic effect.

While the concept of satisfying hunger seems simple enough, we often don't respond to it due to our rigid dieting beliefs. If we don't eat in response to hunger, we remain hungry. If we do eat, we experience guilt. Guilt takes the place of satiation and fosters a negative reinforcement cycle, creating a lose-lose situation.

Feeling positively about the food we eat indicates an alignment in our Body Harmony System. Feeling upset about what we eat indicates a fractured system. Guilt over our eating choices increases this misalignment, while acceptance bridges the gap.

Guilt over past actions creates anxiety over future actions. This starts the rumination process, increasing our experience of hunger. **Simply stated, guilt increases hunger.**

Even though we know the detrimental effects that guilt has on our relationship with food, our actions and ourselves, we are unable to give ourselves a break. Why can't we give up guilt? We would feel too guilty.

The truth is that there is absolutely no benefit to feeling guilty about what we have eaten in the past. We need to replace guilt with the knowledge that living without it will actually minimize hunger and the ensuing run-on eating that it causes. **We need to transform guilt into acceptance and fight it with positive reinforcement. We need to learn to live guilt-free, not fat free.** People often dabble in guilt-free eating and claim that it is not effective. It is not a one-time reprieve that our "selves" are seeking, it is full acceptance of our actions.

NEGATIVE CYCLE	POSITIVE CYCLE
Guilt about past consumption causes anxiety about future consumption. It causes us to ruminate about what we have eaten and what we will eat.	Accepting what we have eaten allows us to stop thinking about food.
The more we ruminate about food, the more the appetite is stimulated and the more hunger we experience.	The less we ruminate about food, the less the appetite is stimulated and the less hunger we experience.

The more hunger we experience, the more we are likely to respond to it by eating or by feeling deprived.	The less hunger we experience, the easier it will be to respond to it in a positive manner.
Eating causes guilt and the cycle repeats itself. (Loop #1)	Positively reinforcing what we have eaten allows us to accept our choices and the cycle repeats itself.
Feeling deprived causes us to ruminate about food and the cycle repeats itself. (Loop #2)	Positively reinforcing what we have eaten allows us to accept our choices and the cycle repeats itself.

GOAL: Learn to live guilt-free.

BOTTOM LINE: Refusing to torment ourselves with feelings of guilt will ultimately minimize hunger, run-on eating and run-on restricting.

8. **Giving ourselves the essential elements of food, water and sleep will maximize our metabolism, making our relationship with food easier to manage.**

8a) **Giving the body the right amount of food when it needs it will boost and/or repair the metabolism to the greatest extent possible, making weight maintenance more manageable.**

When talking about diets and weight maintenance, we often fail to take our metabolism into account. Our metabolism controls the amount of energy our bodies need to survive. It converts the fuel that our bodies need from food into usable energy or stores it in body tissues. When our metabolism is maximized, we convert more food into energy. When our metabolism is impaired, we do not utilize the food that we take in as effectively. As a result, the body needs less to maintain its size. A healthy metabolism will therefore increase the amount of food that we can use making our weight relationship easier to manage.

Physiologically, offering the right amount of nutrients to the body on a timely basis lets the body know that there is enough food to fuel its needs. When the body does not receive the proper nutrients, it assumes that it needs to conserve energy and the metabolism starts to slow down. Failing to respond accurately to Chemical Hunger on a regular basis will negatively affect the metabolism and actually cause the body to require less energy, making weight loss and/or maintenance more difficult and gaining weight easier to achieve.

Psychologically, refusing to respond to hunger tells the mind that something is wrong. The mind will begin to distrust itself and its ability to give the body what it needs, creating a split between the self and the appetite. This dissonance or "separation anxiety" causes the psychological desire for food at times when the body does not need it. It is the opposite of the alignment that we are seeking.

Responding to hunger in a timely basis is the only way to convince the mind and the body that it will be nourished and fed, meaning that there will be no physical or psychological reason for the body to store fuel.

NEGATIVE CYCLE	POSITIVE CYCLE
Failing to respond to Chemical Hunger impairs the metabolism.	Responding to Chemical Hunger maximizes the metabolism.
A reduced metabolism makes weight control and maintenance more difficult to achieve.	Maximizing the metabolism makes weight control and maintenance easier to achieve.
The more difficult our Body Maintenance System, the more restrictive we feel we need to be.	The easier our Body Maintenance System, the less restrictive we feel we need to be.

The more restrictive we feel we need to be, the less likely we are to respond to Chemical Hunger. And the cycle repeats itself.	The less restrictive we feel we need to be, the more likely we are to respond to physical hunger. And the cycle repeats itself.

8b) Adequate sleep and hydration minimizes hunger, clarifies the appetite and enhances the metabolism, making our relationship with food easier to manage.

Sleep, water and food are fundamental and essential elements to maintaining our health and well-being. Without them, we will not survive. There is increased evidence that sleep affects our experience of hunger and our metabolism. In our society, not only do we place limits on our intake, but there is increasing pressure to "do more" and consequently sleep less. When sleep deprived, we may eat to stay awake, often craving sugar and/or caffeine to temporarily alleviate exhaustion. However, both will cause a crash once depleted in our system, leading to further hunger and fatigue. Sleep deprivation also causes hormonal changes that detrimentally affect the metabolism, making the whole Body Maintenance System more difficult. To exacerbate this problem, we make poorer health choices and have more frustrating life experiences when we are over-tired. Finally, we sleep best when we have eaten properly.

Another factor that can affect our experience of hunger is hydration. Hunger can often be confused with thirst. We are 70% water. Food is not. We can live longer without food than without water. It is actually more important for the body to obtain the necessary fluids than the necessary nutrients.

In our society, people often drink coffee in the morning and wine in the evening. Both of these dehydrate the body. When the body is not properly hydrated, the mind can interpret the experience as hunger.

NEGATIVE CYCLE	POSITIVE CYCLE
Food, sleep and water deprivation adversely affect our metabolism and inhibit our ability to accurately read our appetite.	Adequate food, sleep and water maximizes our metabolism and enhances appetite clarity.
Impaired appetite clarity makes it more difficult to determine whether we are hungry, tired or thirsty.	Appetite clarity makes it easier to determine when we are hungry, tired or thirsty.
When we confuse hunger with thirst and exhaustion, it is more difficult to give ourselves what we need.	When we accurately read hunger, exhaustion and thirst, we can respond accordingly.
Responding inaccurately to thirst, hunger and exhaustion is likely to lead to further experiences of deprivation and the cycle repeats itself.	Responding accurately to thirst, hunger and exhaustion allows the body to be satiated, rested and hydrated and the cycle repeats itself.

GOAL: To make our relationship with food easier to manage.

BOTTOM LINE: Offering ourselves sufficient food, water and sleep maximizes our metabolism, making our relationship with food easier to manage.

9. **To be content, we need to balance the effort we put into, and the satisfaction that we obtain from, our Body Maintenance System.**

When following a rigid dieting path, we put so much effort into maintaining our physique that we begin to have unrealistic expectations. This makes it significantly more difficult to become satisfied with the results. To make matters worse, a perceptual disorder can develop where we do not accurately perceive our physical form.

balance the equation and increase our level of satisfaction, we must either put less effort into the process or obtain more fulfillment from it. Body Harmony is achieved when this system is in alignment. As this system becomes more balanced and easier to maintain, we are able to engage in a more natural way of living and being.

NEGATIVE CYCLE	POSITIVE CYCLE
The more difficult our Body Maintenance System, the more effort we must put into the process.	The easier our Body Maintenance System, the less effort we need to put into the process.
The more effort we put into maintaining our bodies, the more we will expect.	The less effort we need to put into maintaining our bodies, the less we will expect.
The more we expect, the harsher we will judge the results.	The less we expect, the more generously we will judge the results.
The harsher we judge the results, the less content we will be.	The more leniently we judge the results, the more content we will be.
The less content we are, the more likely we will be to try to change our bodies.	The more content we are, the less likely we will be to try to change our bodies.
The more likely we are to try to change our bodies, the more effort we will put into the process and the cycle repeats itself.	The less likely we are to try to change our bodies, the less effort we will put into the process and the cycle repeats itself.

GOAL: To have an effortless and natural relationship with food, our bodies and ourselves; to maximize our level of contentment with food, our bodies and ourselves.

BOTTOM LINE: The less effort we put into our Body Maintenance System, the more realistically we will judge ourselves and the more lenient and accepting we will be.

Summary Phase I

When we start to diet due to the critical feelings we have about ourselves, a negative feedback system is created that causes the whole Body Maintenance System to be more difficult than it needs to be. This diet mentality actually fuels our physical and psychological food addictions, separating us from our "self" and causing our behaviours to spiral downward in a seemingly uncontrollable fashion. If we reverse this relationship and create a positive feedback system with food, our bodies and ourselves, we would begin to spiral upwards, synergy would replace depletion, and future possibilities would be endless. What follows is a summary of the negative and positive spiraling cycles. If we look at the overall mechanism in place, we can clearly see what we are doing to ourselves.

NEGATIVE CYCLE	POSITIVE CYCLE
Dieting causes us to restrict our natural eating instincts and separates us from our true appetite.	Responding to our natural eating instincts aligns us with our true appetite.
The less accurately we can respond to our appetite, the less satisfying and efficient eating will be.	The more accurately we can respond to our appetite, the more satisfying and efficient eating will be.
The less satisfied we are from eating, the more we will ruminate about food.	The more satisfied we are from eating, the less we will ruminate about food.
The more we ruminate about food, the more hunger we will experience. The more hunger we experience, the more we will eat. The more we eat, the more guilt we will experience, and the more we will restrict.	Reducing the time spent ruminating about food will reduce the amount of hunger we experience. The less hunger we experience, the easier it will be to respond to it.

Failing to give the body what it needs, when it needs it, (over or under-eating) reduces the effectiveness of the metabolism.	By responding accurately to our appetite, (Pure Essence Eating) the metabolism is maximized to the full extent possible.
The less effective the metabolism, the more difficult it will be to maintain one's weight.	The more effective the metabolism, the easier it will be to maintain a healthy weight.
The more difficult our Body Maintenance System, the more effort we will need to put into weight maintenance.	The easier our Body Maintenance System, the less effort we will need to put into weight maintenance.
The more effort we put into diet and weight maintenance, the more "perfect" we will expect our bodies to be.	The less effort we put into diet and weight maintenance, the less "perfect" we will expect our bodies to be.
The more "perfect" we expect our bodies to be, the less content we will be with them.	The less "perfect" we expect our bodies to be, the more content we will be with them.
The less content we are with our bodies, the more likely we are to engage in disruptive eating patterns. And the cycle repeats itself.	The more content we are with our body, the more likely we are to engage in Pure Essence Eating. And the cycle repeats itself.

The exact order or wording of these steps is not important. The main premise is simple. Dieting separates us from ourselves and makes maintaining our bodies an unnatural and difficult process. When we start to diet because of a negative thought about how we look, we easily fall into a negative feedback system that is psychologically and physically reinforced by negative experiences. It doesn't matter how much weight we gain or lose, the weight maintenance system is more arduous and unpleasant than it needs to be. Even if we physically reach our desired results, we can't enjoy them because our eyes become crueler and focus on only those aspects of our bodies that we are not satisfied with. We learn to live in a constant state of fear, where we worry that any weight loss achieved may be only temporary.

It is easier to follow along our current path. It is easier to fall down the stairs than to walk up. While initially it will take a more concerted effort to change direction, we will come to realize just how much energy we have been losing by our negative state and how much more uplifted we can become by engaging in a positive frame of mind.

To change the direction of this cycle, we must start by thinking positive thoughts about the self and by reaching a point of pure self-acceptance. This process is described in the next section, Phase II.

CYCLE PHASE I

BY GIVING OUR BODY WHAT IT NEEDS WHEN IT NEEDS IT, WE OPTIMIZE OUR RELATIONSHIP WITH FOOD, OUR METABOLISM AND GAIN APPETITE CLARITY TO THE GREATEST EXTENT POSSIBLE.

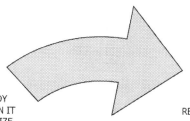

BY OPTIMIZING OUR RELATIONSHIP WITH FOOD, OUR METABOLISM AND GAINING APPETITE CLARITY, WE ARE MORE EASILY ABLE TO GIVE OUR BODY WHAT IT NEEDS WHEN IT NEEDS IT.

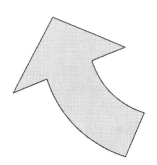

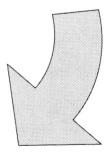

AND THE CYCLE REPEATS ITSELF

The Bottom Line Phase I

```
                    Goal
                   Ph.I: To
                  optimize our
                  relationship
                   with food.


           BOTTOM LINE PHASE I: ENGAGING IN
           PURE ESSENCE EATING ALLOWS US
          TO OPTIMIZE OUR RELATIONSHIP WITH
                         FOOD.


       CONCLUSION PHASE I: THE REALIZATION THAT WE CAN LIVE
      IN ALGINMENT WITH OUR APPETITE IS THE MOST POWERFUL
                  REALIZATION WE WILL HAVE.
```

THE BOTTOM LINE: To optimize our relationship with food we need to give our body what it needs when it needs it. The only way to determine what the body needs is to consult the appetite. The only way to improve our ability to read our appetite is to rely on it over externally derived rules. The less time we spend thinking, fretting, planning, strategizing and scheming about food, the less hunger we will experience and the clearer our appetite will be. The more we positively reinforce our actions by sending positive messages to ourselves, the more likely we will be to trust our appetite and strengthen our connection to it. The more we focus on our experiences of hunger in the present moment, the better we will be able to accurately respond to them. The less guilt we allow ourselves to feel, the less hunger we will experience. Giving ourselves the essential elements of food, water and rest will maximize our metabolism, making our weight maintenance system easier to manage. The less effort we put into our weight maintenance system, the more realistically we will judge the results and the more lenient and accepting we will be.

The Bye-Cycle Wheel Phase I

THROUGH REACHING OUR GOALS, THE BYE-CYCLE WHEEL MOVES US FORWARD AND TRANSPORTS US TO A NEW WAY OF LIVING.....TO A NEW WAY OF PERCEIVING, EXPERIENCING AND RESPONDING TO HUNGER.

NEGATIVE CYCLE   POSITIVE CYCLE

GOALS PHASE I

By accurately experiencing, interpreting and responding to our natural appetite, we will be able to rely on it to tell us what and when we need to eat, clarifying our experience of hunger. We can strengthen our relationship with our appetite by offering ourselves positive thoughts surrounding our responses to hunger. By aligning hunger with desire and learning to live guilt-free, we will make our relationship with food easier to manage. Ultimately, we can have an effortless and natural relationship with food, our bodies and ourselves.

Phase Two: Self-Acceptance

In Phase I, we have come to understand the path that dieters can take and how it leads to a self-perpetuating downward spiral of thoughts, energy and actions. We can change the direction of our cycle from negative to positive by using our own personal GPS system. By following a **Guided Psychological State,** we can give ourselves the **Gift of Personal and Physiological Synergy** and allow ourselves to capitalize on our own personal power. To do this, we need to guide our thoughts to create a **purely positive psychological state** that can give us the stability and the grounding we need to rise up. While it will initially take additional effort to consciously change the way we think, once we change our "de-synergistic" cycle to a "synergistic" one, we will have all the energy we need to continue along our new path.

In Phase I, we discussed the functional aspects of our eating behaviours. In Phase II, we focus on the psychological aspects of the mind. Once again we rely on *The Laws of Gravity* to assist us on our journey.

10. Weight loss achieved as a result of self-loathing will result in self-loathing. Weight loss achieved as a result of self-acceptance will result in self-acceptance.

If we start a diet through lack of self-acceptance, we will never truly be able to accept ourselves regardless of the physical outcome. To force ourselves to diet because we dislike our bodies, creates a detrimental negative feedback cycle. We teach ourselves to fear what our appetites and our bodies will do, separating instead of aligning us with our Natural State. Unfortunately, when we are on this destructive path, there is no magical point where we are allowed to feel reassured. Even if we reach our weight loss goal, the "success" is short-lived because we have put conditions on our self-acceptance. Instead of celebrating, we learn to live in constant fear of falling out of favour with ourselves if we regain or cease to lose more weight.

We fully believe that we will be able to accept ourselves once we reach a certain weight. This is rarely the case, due to the Perceptual Distortion that accompanies eating disturbances. It causes us to judge our achievements and physique more harshly even when weight loss is achieved. This is where our Self-Concept merges with our Body Image. The negative feelings that we have about ourselves, pre-weight loss, are projected onto the mirror throughout our dieting journey. We distort our physical form and view ourselves as being quite different from our actual size and shape. When we look at past pictures of ourselves, we can often see how out of touch our body image was with our physical reality.

If the goal of dieting is to feel good about ourselves, and we start off feeling favourably, then we are in alignment with our goal. If we start off with a negative self-concept, we are at odds with our goal. If we need to lose weight to redeem ourselves, we are putting a great deal of pressure on ourselves to stay on the diet and for the diet to be successful, thus embarking on an extremely difficult journey. This added stress makes the whole process much harder to follow and to maintain.

It is also true that when we feel good about ourselves, we are likely to have an intrinsic desire to put healthy, nourishing food into our bodies and to lead a healthy lifestyle. We tend to have a realistic and positive self-image. If we start the dieting process by feeling badly about ourselves, we are less inclined to treat our bodies well. We are more likely to try to trick our bodies and to try to get away with destructive behaviours when the mood strikes us or to engage in black and white thinking, which leads to "purely good" or "purely bad" cycles of yo-yo dieting.

GOAL: To start our journey by offering ourselves unconditional self-acceptance instead of expecting to accept ourselves at some "perfect point" in the future.

BOTTOM LINE: The more we focus on losing weight as a means of achieving self-acceptance, the more difficult losing weight will be. When we accept ourselves, we are more likely to treat ourselves well and to engage in a healthy lifestyle.

11. Self-acceptance is the only way to positively move forward.

Boosting our internal psychological state by engaging in self-acceptance is the only way out of our detrimental way of relating to ourselves. By starting in a positive place, we can use our Personal GPS system and Guide our Psychological State to generate encouraging thoughts surrounding food and our bodies. **Self-acceptance is the soil (soul) in which the seed of a healthy relationship with food can take root and grow.**

There are many different levels and aspects of self-acceptance. There is the acceptance of our bodies, our dieting history, our genetic make-up and, of course, our eating. Individuals who start dieting from a place of negativity often dismiss their dieting history and blame themselves for their genetic make-up. They feel that they cannot fully accept their eating behaviours because they believe that self-critical thoughts are what keep them from being "bad". They fail to realize that it is the negative thinking itself that creates the disharmony within the self and makes a very natural process, such as hunger, so difficult to manage.

The truth is that all past actions are history and cannot be altered. In the present moment we cannot change what we have eaten, our dieting history, our bodies, our metabolism or our weight. There is therefore absolutely no benefit to be derived from harshly judging anything that we have done. Since we cannot change our past and feeling guilty is detrimental to the self, the most beneficial thing that we can do in any one moment in time is to **accept.** It matters not what our actions are but whether or not we are able to make peace with them. It is the simple act of **acceptance** that will serve us well. This is what we have given up on our dieting path and what we need to reclaim. The more we can **accept** our actions and their repercussions in the present, the better equipped we will be to repeat the process and the brighter our futures will be.

We must therefore learn to accept every single one of our actions leading up to this very second. This includes what we have put ourselves through and the effect that it has had on our bodies and our minds. Finally, the more readily we can accept our actions, the greater confidence we will have in ourselves and the easier it will be to continue to validate our choices….and the cycle will repeat itself. The more time we spend second guessing ourselves, the less confidence we will have and the more likely we will be to question our actions….and the cycle repeats itself.

It can be extremely difficult to stop negative thinking even though we may be aware of its detrimental effects. Initially, it will be necessary to apply an equal or greater force to change the psychological direction or pattern of our thoughts. As this system is primarily unconscious, we will need to use conscious effort to do this.

GOAL: Accepting all past actions.

THE BOTTOM LINE: Our future actions are more likely to be positive when we accept our past actions. Guilt about past actions is of no benefit to us.

12. Self-acceptance can only occur in the moment and is an on-going dynamic activity, not a permanent state.

For people with eating issues, there is a frustrating gap between our experiences and our Natural State. Our Natural State represents the relationship that we would have had with food, our metabolisms, our bodies and ourselves had our eating patterns never been disrupted. To bridge this gap, we need to accept where we are in our journey right now. By doing so, we will connect with ourselves to the greatest extent possible and continue to move towards a more natural way of being, travelling on the most positive path we can follow. We are acting within our Natural State when we offer ourselves unconditional acceptance and do not expect ourselves to be anywhere else on our journey than where we are at this particular moment. Each moment of acceptance will bring us closer to our Natural State.

There is no future or past to self-acceptance. The process of positive or negative thinking can only occur in the moment and can change from one second to the next. Each positive thought brings us closer in alignment with our Natural State. Each negative thought takes us further away. The difference between spiraling up and spiraling down starts with one single positive thought. We have to keep making this conscious switch to positive thoughts as many times as necessary. If a negative thought slips in, we must remember that the very next thought can be one of acceptance. The shift will become easier as the positive spiraling gains momentum. Remember, just as we can spiral downward in a seemingly out of control fashion (de-synergize), we can spiral upward into a manageable state (synergy).

Some of us might try to attempt this shift to positive thinking through the use of a strict or disciplined approach. However, getting out of the negative spiral actually requires the opposite type of behavior, giving ourselves a break. "Slipping up" is not something to be feared because it is simply the next action that we have to accept. It is not the behavior that is important, but the thoughts that surround it. The way that we view and react to our past actions will determine the direction of the cycle that we follow, not the actions themselves. The process at play here is significantly more important than the actual behaviours.

We must embark on this journey without expecting it to be perfect or that we will reach some ideal state. Our focus cannot be on the destination, but on the journey itself. We must not be fooled into believing that changing who we are will make us happy. There is no guarantee that we will be content with ourselves in the future, if we fail to be satisfied with ourselves in the present. The future is a culmination of each present moment and therefore cannot be any different, any better or any worse, than the series of moments leading up to it. Creating the most pleasant "nows" will ultimately give us the best possible outcome.

GOAL: To be in as close an alignment with our Natural State (pre-disrupted state) as possible.

BOTTOM LINE: By treating ourselves with respect, caring and understanding, regardless of the behaviours we exhibit, we will be as close as we can be to our Natural State.

13. We can only experience hunger in the moment.

Just as self-acceptance can occur only in the moment, hunger is a present moment phenomenon. We cannot experience past or future hunger. Yet, as dieters, we spend a great deal of time thinking about what we have eaten in the past and what we will eat in the future. What we have had for lunch often determines what we will allow ourselves to have for dinner and our current state of hunger is often ignored. Any guilt over past meals makes us apprehensive about our next ones. Contemplation of future eating causes anxiety, as we fear that we will not be able to live up to our "dieting expectations". All this ruminating about past and future meals simply serves to increase our experience of hunger. These exaggerated levels of desire dissolve when we focus on tuning into our appetite in the present moment. Strategically, our best plan is to positively reinforce all past actions and then stop thinking about them, minimizing any run-on thoughts about food. If we respond to current hunger requests with positive messages of abundance ("I can have what I need."), we won't have to fret or worry about what we will have in the future because we will be confident that we will be able to satisfy our hunger when it arises.

To stop thinking about food in the moment, we need to give ourselves enough nutrients to satiate our body and calm the mind. We need to respond to hunger in a way that we can accept without guilt or self-criticism. We must make peace with our eating decisions and respond in the best way that we can in the moment. We need to learn to MASTER Pure Essence Eating for Creative Eaters (MASTERPEECE). Eventually, if we give up the negative retribution and the resulting downward spiraling, we will have greater appetite clarity. We will experience less Phantom Hunger and will need to respond only to Chemical Hunger. But, until then, we must respond to any form of hunger that we experience with grace, patience and consideration. In fact, we need to be even more understanding when we are having difficulty clarifying our hunger. At these times we can, once again, consciously use our personal GPS system, to Guide our internal Psychological State to make certain that our thoughts and our eating experiences remain positive and constructive.

GOAL: Think only about hunger in the moment.

BOTTOM LINE: Focusing only on our actual experiences of hunger, without reference to past or future eating, makes the whole Body Maintenance System easier. Guilt and anxiety surrounding past or future eating makes the whole process unnecessarily difficult.

14. **We win the battle by changing our experience of hunger, not by suppressing it.**

Fighting with hunger is a battle that cannot be won. By changing our experience of hunger, we cannot lose.

Our goal is not to fight with hunger, it is to change our experience of it. We do not need to force ourselves to put down food or to deny our hunger. That is simply part of the inner struggle that feeds our eating issues and separates us from our Natural State. Hunger is not the enemy, it is our ally. If we are able to fully and clearly experience hunger as it naturally occurs in alignment with our appetite, we will be able to determine exactly what our body needs. When we give our body exactly what it needs and are able to respond positively to its requests, we won't have to fight with food because we won't have to manipulate the way we eat.

GOAL: To ensure that our experiences of hunger are in line with our true appetite.

BOTTOM LINE: The best chance we have of changing the way we experience hunger is by attempting to align ourselves with our appetite and positively reinforcing our attempts.

15. **Only by wanting what we currently have, can we guarantee our contentment.**

Desiring what we do not have guarantees our dissatisfaction. Getting what we do not have (what we think we want) does not actually guarantee anything.

It is human nature to want what we can't have and to create an idealistic illusion around that which is not in our possession. Whether it is food, money, a relationship, or weight loss, that which is outside of our reach is unrealistically alluring.

However, there is absolutely no guarantee that getting what we want will bring us any more satisfaction than we are currently able to experience. The future is an unknown that we can't ever enjoy now. We can only enjoy it when it gets here. However, coveting what we do not have is certain to cause unhappiness and dissatisfaction now. Therefore, to "lock in" our happiness and contentment, we need to focus on our accepting our present state.

As dieters, we are future oriented and often dismiss our present state because we are not content with it. We try to change what we don't like about ourselves, and/or our bodies and/or our lives by dieting. Since dieting does not fix all areas of our lives, we are left disappointed and turn back to the diet and to weight loss to miraculously solve all our problems. Even though we know this process is not effective, we continue along the same path, with the same goal, experiencing more and more frustration along the way. We then blame our unhappiness on our dieting failure or if successful in our dieting efforts, we raise the bar and set a new physical goal for ourselves. This ensures that we will never have what we "want", because our "want" changes along the way. This process causes us to feel bad about ourselves and we simply turn back to the diet to resolve our concerns.

Dieting offers us perceived control over our appearance. However, to a great extent, we don't have control over our physical form. Our bodies have a fundamental genetic makeup which determines our general shape and cannot be altered through diet. Dieting cannot change our hair colour, our height or our facial features. While a good haircut and flattering clothes often make a bigger difference than a few pounds, we often forego the hairdresser to get to the gym and wear baggy clothes that hide our shape.

Even though most dieting efforts do not result in permanent physical transformations, we continue to diet, with that goal in mind. Since transforming our external selves won't solve all of our problems and since we can't change our external selves in the present moment, the best thing we can do now is to accept where we are. If we expect to change what we cannot alter (in the moment), we are doomed to experience disappointment and frustration. If we expect to change ourselves in the future, we are destined to dislike ourselves in the present.

If our initial goal is inner peace and contentment, then it would be most beneficial to align our goal with what is readily available to us so that we can have positive experiences now. **We need to practice self-acceptance so that we can master it.** If we can learn to accept what we have within our reach, and enjoy each part of our journey, then we will have reached our goal. The truth is that if we do end up changing our shape in the future, the journey from "here" to "there" will be easier and more enjoyable if we are able to practice self-acceptance.

This is not a diet book and should not be followed with an expectation of weight loss, weight gain or weight maintenance. Such expectations lead to anticipation of the future and will only act as a trigger, potentially causing a downward spinning cycle of rumination, hunger and anxiety.

It's not about being a specific size. It's about being comfortable being the size we are. We do not have to reshape our bodies to attain inner peace and contentment. We need to reshape our minds and let our bodies take care of themselves. We need to give up control over the pace of our recovery, over our hunger and our weight and take charge of our intra-psychic responses and ultimately, how we relate to ourselves.

GOAL: Align our expectations with what is currently within our grasp so that we can obtain more moments of inner peace and contentment.

BOTTOM LINE: If we are at peace and are content right now, then we have reached our goal.

16. The most important commitment that we can make is to "not abandon ourselves".

Relate, don't alienate.

The real fear that we have about staying on a diet is **not** whether we can achieve and maintain weight loss, but what our minds will do to us throughout the process. If we prove that we will support, not alienate (alien-ate) ourselves, we will have nothing to fear from external factors. Our external appearance, our mirror image, and our weight will have no power over us if our minds refuse to turn against us.

A secondary gain refers to the underlying benefit of a process. Negative thoughts about the self are a secondary gain of eating disturbances. We can feel upset at ourselves and avoid dealing with more difficult issues if we constantly focus on food. If the subconscious goal of our "creative eating patterns" is to feel bad about who we are, and we refuse to feel bad, the process will no longer work. We will actually eliminate the need to have the problem in the first place.

GOAL: To prove to ourselves that we will not turn against ourselves.

BOTTOM LINE: External factors have no power over us if we internally support ourselves.

17. Only we can determine what our body needs and when it needs it.

As dieters, we separate ourselves from our appetites, actually fearing it and deeming hunger to be the enemy. Because of this, we rarely know when we are hungry, when we are full or what type of nutrition we need. Of our own volition, we give our power to an external set of rules and choose to live in a state of perceived powerlessness. By following a diet, and listening to an outside source, we basically abdicate responsibility for accurately reading and responding to our hunger and focus on whether or not we can stick to a diet. We fail to respond to our internal experiences or judge whether the diet has effectively allowed us to manage and respond to our hunger. When we are unable to stick to the diet, we blame ourselves, not the diet, for our failure.

Figuring out what our body wants, when it wants it, can be a huge undertaking that comes with a very long learning curve. While this process should not be belittled, it should be emphasized that we are the only ones who can go through it. We are the only ones who can read our hunger, who can determine what type of food is satiating and what type leaves us hungry. While others can offer all types of information regarding nutrition, only we can know what we are experiencing. No other person, regardless of how knowledgeable, can monitor our internal state.

We are Dorothy and are all wearing the red ruby slippers (or top-siders), known as the appetite, which we can rely on to guide us. Intrinsically, we know this. These words are simply a reminder of who we are. To successfully deal with our eating behaviours, we must create an eating regime that conforms to our needs as opposed to conforming to a diet. We have to figure out a method that works for us. We have to own it and take responsibility for it.

Dieting creates perceived powerlessness over how we eat. Yet, under no circumstances, on or off a diet, are we actually under another's control. Eating is our choice. Choosing the diet over "us" gives our power away and ultimately undermines the relationship that we have with ourselves.

It is time to take our power back. Remember, no one has actually taken it from us. We have given it of our own free will. Still, it will take determination and resilience to re-claim it. This internal strength and self-honesty will support the type of relationship that we must develop with ourselves on our journey out of the "diet zone".

GOAL: Accept the responsibility for accurately reading our appetite; to establish an internal path for interpreting and responding to hunger.

THE BOTTOM LINE: We are the only ones who can determine our state of hunger.

18. Healed perfectly is not perfectly healed.

Many people feel that they will accept themselves when they are "perfectly healed". While dieting, this requires reaching an "ideal weight". When attempting to end the dieting cycle, this refers to being completely free from disrupted eating behaviours.

We must be careful about attempts to become "perfectly healed" as this may generate the same negative judgments that dieting has created in the past. While there is no such thing as a "perfect state", we can enter a more "naturally dynamic" one. Instead of thinking in black and white, we can learn to live in the gray zone. Wherever we are at in our healing journey, we can start now taking one small step upward at a time. By accepting our inability to be "perfectly healed", we are able to create a more positive relationship with ourselves now and as we move forward.

The Laws of Gravity have been broken down into individual steps to enable us to find one small step that we can climb at a time. The more stairs we go up, the easier it will be to keep rising. While it is not realistic to think that we are going to be perfectly in sync with our appetite from this moment forward, it is possible for us to refuse to turn on ourselves or to feel guilty when we are not. Even if we cannot choose the right meal, we can accept and positively reinforce our choice as the best decision we could have made at time. Even if we cannot give up our dieting rules, we may be able to override one of them. We may be able to turn diet restrictions into guidelines that can assist us in responding to our appetite instead of preventing us from doing so. Even if we can't change our eating patterns immediately, we can give ourselves more sleep and stay better hydrated. We can try to look at food as being abundant instead of a scarce resource. We can look at our appetite as our ally instead of our enemy. We can look for "moments of appetite clarity" and focus on the times when we get it right, when we respond accurately to our appetite and are able to get a glimpse of what our lives could be like. We can have faith that with full acceptance of our journey and our efforts, in time, these moments will become days, weeks and a way of life. We can try to create an internally driven energy system whereby we take more responsibility for our decisions and stop giving power over to external rules. We can start accepting our actions and offering ourselves praise instead of criticism. We need to do this as quickly or as slowly as necessary in order to take safe, solid steps forward and upward. We must be mindful not to judge the process and absolutely refuse to turn on the self.

GOAL: Rise upward on our path, climbing as many steps as we are able; to acknowledge and appreciate any progress we have made on our journey.

BOTTOM LINE: Any affirmative action we take, regardless of how small or individually insignificant, will change the direction of the route that we follow from a descending to an ascending one.

CYCLE PHASE II

BY ENGAGING IN PURE SELF-ACCEPTANCE, WE MAKE THE SHIFT FROM A DE-SYNERGISTIC NEGATIVE CYCLE TO A SYNERGISTIC POSITIVE ONE.

WHEN POSITIVELY SPIRALING UPWARD, IT IS EASIER TO ACCEPT THE SELF.

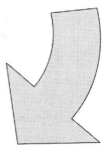

AND THE CYCLE REPEATS ITSELF

The Bottom Line Phase II

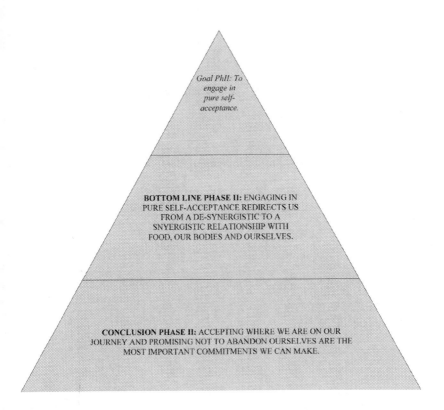

Goal PhII: To engage in pure self-acceptance.

BOTTOM LINE PHASE II: ENGAGING IN PURE SELF-ACCEPTANCE REDIRECTS US FROM A DE-SYNERGISTIC TO A SNYERGISTIC RELATIONSHIP WITH FOOD, OUR BODIES AND OURSELVES.

CONCLUSION PHASE II: ACCEPTING WHERE WE ARE ON OUR JOURNEY AND PROMISING NOT TO ABANDON OURSELVES ARE THE MOST IMPORTANT COMMITMENTS WE CAN MAKE.

The more we focus on losing weight as a means of achieving self-acceptance, the more difficult losing weight will be. We can make the Body Maintenance System easier to manage by focusing on our actual experiences of hunger, without reference to past or future eating. However, feeling guilty or anxious about what we have or will eat makes the whole process unnecessarily difficult. We don't need to fight with hunger, we need to clarify it. The best chance we have of doing this is by tuning into our appetite, for we are the only ones who can determine our internal state of hunger. We need to positively reinforce any attempts that we make regardless of the eating patterns we exhibit. By treating ourselves with respect, caring and understanding, we are more likely to naturally treat ourselves well and to engage in a healthy lifestyle. Future actions are much more likely to be constructive, when we start off in a positive place of acceptance. The truth is, if we are internally supportive, external factors such as weight and body image will have no power over us. And any affirmative action we take, regardless of how small or individually insignificant, will change the direction of the route that we follow from a descending to an ascending one. One final note, if we start the whole process being at peace with ourselves, then in many ways, we will have already reached our goal.

The Bye-Cycle Wheel Phase II

THROUGH REACHING OUR GOALS, THE BYE-CYCLE WHEEL MOVES US FORWARD AND TRANSPORTS US TO A NEW WAY OF LIVING.....TO A NEW WAY OF PERCEIVING, EXPERIENCING AND RESPONDING TO HUNGER.

NEGATIVE CYCLE   POSITIVE CYCLE

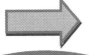

GOALS PHASE II

Start our journey by offering ourselves unconditional self-acceptance instead of expecting to accept ourselves in the future. This means accepting ALL past actions so that we can be in as close an alignment with our Natural State (pre-disrupted state) as possible. Instead of fighting with hunger, we want to change our experience of it so that we can think about food only in the moments when we need it. If we align our expectations with what is currently within our grasp, we will be able to obtain more moments of inner peace and contentment. By self-supporting and self-promoting, we will be able to take whatever steps we need to rise upward on our path, acknowledging and appreciating any progress we have made on our journey. By accepting the responsibility for accurately reading our appetite, we will be able to establish an internal path for interpreting and responding to hunger.

Phase Three: Allow

In Phase I, we have come to understand the path that we, as dieters take, and how it leads to a self-perpetuating downward spiral of thoughts, energy and actions. In Phase II, we learned that self-acceptance can assist us in redirecting our path from negative to positive cycling and that this can alter our internal experiences of hunger and improve our relationship with food. In Phase III, we focus on our internal emotional state and the affect that this has on our relationship with ourselves.

19. **If we neglect our internal emotional state, it will impact the clarity of our appetite and alter our experience of hunger.**

Outwardly Good....Inwardly Bad.

For chronic dieters, our emotional state is intricately tied to our experience of hunger and our resulting eating behaviours. An eating disturbance is a coping mechanism that is used to avoid dealing with how we feel. Eating disturbances separate us from our emotions by causing us to focus on eating instead of the issues being ignored. Initially, they actually work as an effective avoidance strategy. However, when issues remain unresolved they become exponentially bigger. Hence, the eating disturbance must become much worse in order to continue to escape dealing with our emotional concerns.

The more concerns we bury, the more energy we need to spend to keep them hidden. The whole process spirals downward, taking on momentum. As we continue to neglect our problems, we remain preoccupied with what we have eaten. We focus on our external bodies instead of our internal state; hiding and negating any aspects of ourselves that we feel are undesirable so that we can portray a favourable image to the world.

Burying these feelings and thoughts with food seems to be the only way we can feel okay about ourselves. Eventually, anything that is deemed unacceptable gets pushed down and internalized, creating a negative internal state. The worse we feel inside, the greater the pressure to display a positive exterior and conceal our true internal climate from others and ourselves. Hiding is a key aspect of this problem which is why eating disturbances thrive in solitude and separate us from ourselves and others. Ultimately, this creates a split within the self and the dissonance leaves people feeling isolated, at odds with themselves, and wondering why the process has become so unbearably difficult.

As Chemical Hunger is not pervasive enough to distract us all of the time, we need to find something that will take over our thoughts continuously. Since Phantom Hunger isn't real, it cannot be satisfied and therefore serves as a constant distraction from our internal emotional state. Being distracted prevents us from dealing with our "real issues". We use food to become pervasively numb, and eventually, eating becomes our only way of experiencing emotions. If we want to feel sad or guilty, we will eat something we can feel sad or guilty about. By avoiding how we feel, we learn to feel nothing and end up not being present in our own lives.

Many of us believe that we do want to end our struggles with food but seem to experience some internal resistance that prevents us from doing so. The best kept secret is that on some level, we don't want to give up our "unique eating patterns" as they allow us to "stay safe" and are a secondary gain of eating difficulties. It is much easier to believe that we have a flaw, than to face life without something to blame our struggles on. It is much easier to continue our complicated relationship with food than to live without our coping mechanism. The truth is that when we stop focusing on food, there is nothing keeping these emotions down and the buried pain is free to arise. That is actually when the real work begins, dealing with these unwanted feelings about ourselves that we have neglected. Unfortunately, just as we did not develop the necessary skills to respond to hunger, we have not developed the skills required to identify and respond to our emotional state. When a feeling arises, it is uncomfortable and we are eager to be rid of it. This is when we return to the destructive eating behaviours that we have relied upon in the past, once again, wondering why dieting has become so complicated.

Unfortunately, eating disruptions cause us to feel bad about who we are and separate us from our Natural (pre-disrupted) State. Being disconnected from our internal emotional state causes us to put excess pressure on our external physical state. Eventually, we begin to identify solely with our external bodies and confuse this with our self-worth. To make matters worse, we are living in an appearance and weight obsessed society. Since our eating affects how we look, we are judged by our eating behaviours. Thus, in society's eye, we actually become our eating disturbance! We are graded on this physical form that does not represent who we would be in our Natural State. The truth is that we are not our eating disturbance. How we eat is not the essence of who we are, but simply the behaviours that we engage in. We need to wake up and remind ourselves of this fact. We are born knowing but somewhere along the way we forget and submit to a more deprecating self-concept which causes us unnecessary pain and suffering. We need to become re-aligned with our natural selves and learn to live in a more natural manner, returning to our Natural State.

GOAL: To deal directly with our emotions and prevent them from interfering with our relationship with food.

BOTTOM LINE: Dealing directly with our emotions minimizes the need to use food as a coping mechanism.

20. Our internal emotional state ultimately affects the relationship that we have with ourselves.

It's not about the form, it's about the feeling.

The buried emotions that we have stored throughout out dieting journey detrimentally affect our internal state. Because of this, we see current events through a shaded lens which blurs our view. By cleaning out our emotional reservoir, our sight becomes clearer and our feelings, more relevant to our current experiences. Thus we may alter our inner experiences by dealing with past ones.

It is not likely that we will ever fully unpack our emotional baggage and wipe our past slate clean. There will always be a risk of becoming emotionally flooded in a seemingly innocuous situation. However, the more we exercise our "emotional muscles", the better able we will be to cope with any feelings that arise.

While the details of reuniting with our internal emotional state are beyond the scope of this book and deserve a greater level of attention, the basic premise may be described in the following manner.

We must first create a purely positive psychological state surrounding food and eating. When we do this, we will be able to stop the conscious mind from focusing on food. In the absence of this conscious distraction, the inner emotions that we have buried will be allowed to surface. If we offer ourselves unconditional positive regard and create a safe internal environment, the psyche will allow past issues to rise up into our consciousness. Once emotions have arisen, we need to acknowledge and accept them without judging them, ignoring them, suppressing them or reacting to them. We need to promise not to turn against ourselves for experiencing them. We need to try to understand them for what they are, buried feelings that have long been ignored. If we allow them to be and to last as long as necessary, we will be able to release the pain that we have buried. Not all past emotions have to rise up, but we can be open and accepting of those that do.

The more intra-psychic pain we release without consequence, the more we will trust that we are capable of dealing with our concerns without judging or abandoning ourselves. The less fear we have of experiencing our feelings, the more we will let rise up. The more buried emotions we release, the less negative our internal state will be and the less we will have to hide. And the cycle repeats itself, until ultimately, this type of "self-honesty" sets us free from our de-synergistic relationship with food, our bodies and ourselves.

Since we can only be in the present moment, we can only feel in the present moment. Even though we may remember past experiences and release buried emotions, we can only experience them now, in our current state, at our current age, with our current perspective. As such, we may experience them differently now than we did years ago. How we experience them is not as relevant as the fact that we are experiencing them. **It is about living in a state of feeling, now and from this moment forward.**

A NOTE ON PERSONAL SAFETY: Please note that for some, the experience of these True Emotions may be overwhelming. We need to ensure that we **stay safe** and have a support system in place at all times so that we can deal with the emotions that arise.

NEGATIVE CYCLE	POSITIVE CYCLE
The more we focus on food, the less psychological energy we will have to deal with our emotional state.	The less we focus on food, the more psychological energy we will have to deal with our emotional state.
The less we deal with our emotions, the less we will be able to effectively deal with our concerns.	The more we deal with our emotions, the more we will be able to effectively deal with our concerns.
The less capable we are of dealing with our concerns, the less we will be willing to experience.	The more capable we are of dealing with the concerns, the more emotions we will allow to rise up.
The less we experience, the more emotions we will have to keep buried.	The more we experience, the fewer emotions we will have to bury.
The more emotional baggage we keep buried, the more we will need to rely on food as an emotional distraction. And the cycle repeats itself.	The less emotional baggage we keep buried, the less we will need to rely on food as an emotional distraction. And the cycle repeats itself.

SIMPLY STATED.........

NEGATIVE CYCLE	POSITIVE CYCLE
The more we avoid dealing with our emotions, the more we will need to focus on food as a distraction.	The more directly we deal with our emotions, the less we will need to focus on food.
The more we focus on food, the less we will be able to experience and deal with our emotions. And the cycle repeats itself.	The less we focus on food, the more we will be able to experience and deal with our emotions. And the cycle repeats itself.

20 a) To connect with our internal state, we need to deal with our true underlying emotions as opposed to surface distractions.

Just as we sought to alter our internal experiences of hunger by reconnecting to our appetite, we seek to alter our internal emotional experiences by reconnecting with ourselves.

Many individuals will argue that they deal directly with emotional experiences and self-connect emotionally. We can, in fact, lead what feels like a rather highly charged life without actually experiencing our true feelings. What can be confusing is that there are different types of emotions. In the same way that we can experience both Chemical and Phantom Hunger, we can feel both True and Surface Emotions. While True Emotions allow us to accurately understand how we are feeling, Surface Emotions disguise the underlying issue and create an effective distraction, causing us to use our energy to deal with the drama. Responding to Surface Emotions does not provide us with the release that we need as these emotions are not the root cause of the problem. When we deal with our True Emotions directly, we have the opportunity to correctly address and potentially resolve our troubles. Even if there is nothing that we can do to change a situation, experiencing and releasing True Emotions can create an altered internal state, bringing us closer to our true selves which will ultimately assist us in our healing journey. Instead of judging or reacting to our internal emotional experiences, we seek to simply understand and interpret them better.

We have learned that hunger is not the enemy. It is our ally. If we can experience and respond to Chemical Hunger, we need not reject our requests for food. Experiencing our true emotions is the path to eliminating Phantom Hunger, making our appetite clearer and Chemical Hunger easier to read.

NEGATIVE CYCLE	POSITIVE CYCLE
SURFACE EMOTIONS	TRUE EMOTIONS
Surface Emotions mask what we are really feeling.	True Emotions tell us how we are really feeling.
Responding to Surface Emotions does not solve situations and can create more drama.	Responding to how we are really feeling allows us to deal with our concerns directly.
Focusing on the drama allows us to avoid the underlying issues and prevents us from dealing with what is wrong.	Focusing on our problems allows us to deal with and resolve our issues.
The more time and effort we spend dealing with Surface Emotions, the less energy we will have to deal with our True Emotions and the less connected we will be to how we really feel.	The more time and effort we spend dealing directly with our True Emotions and resolving our problems, the more connected we will be to how we feel.
The less connected we are to how we feel, the more we will focus on the surface drama. And the cycle repeats itself.	The more connected we are to how we really feel, the easier it will be to continue to deal with our True Emotions. And the cycle repeats itself.

GOAL: To experience and deal with our True Emotions; to live in a state of feeling.

BOTTOM LINE: Dealing with our True underlying Emotions eliminates the need to create drama or emotional distractions in our lives.

CYCLE PHASE III

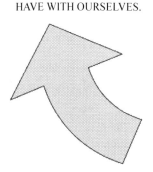

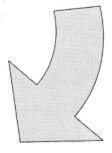

BY EXPERIENCING AND
DEALING DIRECTLY
WITH OUR FEELINGS,
WE ARE ABLE TO GAIN
EMOTIONAL CLARITY
AND OPTIMIZE THE
RELATIONSHIP THAT WE
HAVE WITH OURSELVES.

BY GAINING
EMOTIONAL CLARITY
AND OPTIMIZING OUR
RELATIONSHIP WITH
OURSELVES, WE ARE
ABLE TO EXPERIENCE
AND DEAL DIRECTLY
WITH OUR FEELINGS.

AND THE CYCLE REPEATS
ITSELF

The Bottom Line Phase III

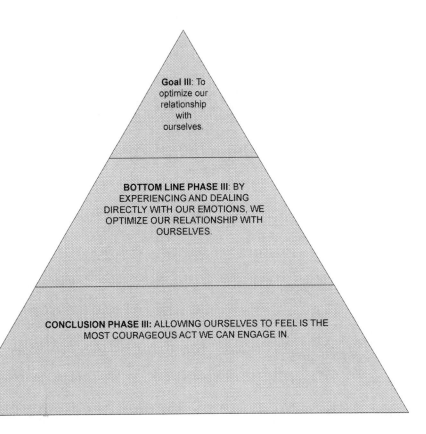

Goal III: To optimize our relationship with ourselves.

BOTTOM LINE PHASE III: BY EXPERIENCING AND DEALING DIRECTLY WITH OUR EMOTIONS, WE OPTIMIZE OUR RELATIONSHIP WITH OURSELVES.

CONCLUSION PHASE III: ALLOWING OURSELVES TO FEEL IS THE MOST COURAGEOUS ACT WE CAN ENGAGE IN.

Dealing with our True underlying Emotions eliminates the need for us to use food to create drama or emotional distractions in our lives.

The Bye-Cycle Wheel Phase III

THROUGH REACHING OUR GOALS, THE BYE-CYCLE WHEEL MOVES US FORWARD AND TRANSPORTS US TO A NEW WAY OF LIVING.....TO A NEW WAY OF PERCEIVING, EXPERIENCING AND RESPONDING TO HUNGER.

NEGATIVE CYCLE   POSITIVE CYCLE

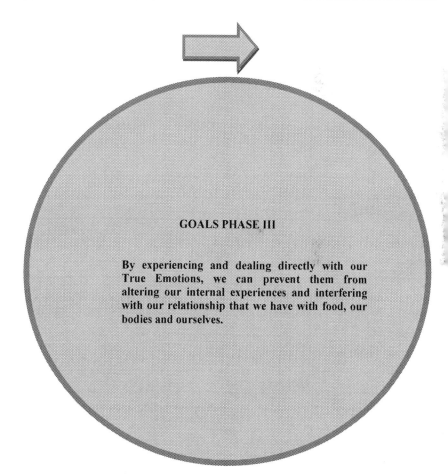

GOALS PHASE III

By experiencing and dealing directly with our True Emotions, we can prevent them from altering our internal experiences and interfering with our relationship that we have with food, our bodies and ourselves.

In Conclusion…..

Re-Align, Don't Resign

In summary, our overall goal is to create a positive, synergistic cycle of relating to food, our bodies, our emotions and ourselves. To do this, we need to re-align with our natural selves and return to our Natural State.

SUMMARY PHASE I
By obtaining appetite clarity, we optimize our relationship with food.
By optimizing our relationship with food, we obtain appetite clarity.
And the cycle repeats itself.

SUMMARY PHASE II
By practicing self-acceptance, we are able to optimize our relationship with food, with our bodies and with ourselves.
By optimizing our relationship with food, with our bodies and with ourselves, it is easier to accept ourselves.
And the cycle repeats itself.

SUMMARY PHASE III
By optimizing our relationship with ourselves, we obtain emotional clarity.
By obtaining emotional clarity, we optimize our relationship with ourselves.
And the cycle repeats itself.

FINAL SUMMARY
Pure essence eating leads to pure essence living.
Pure essence living leads to pure essence eating.
And the cycle repeats itself.

Self-Acceptance is the missing link that allows us to say Good-Bye to a Negative Cycle and start a Positive Cycle of living, giving us the energy and the psychological environment we need to deal with the emotional aspects of ourselves that we have neglected. It allows us to make peace (masterpeece) with our eating history and current behaviours so that we can focus on the more important issues in our lives.

These Laws represent whole truths that we were born knowing but have long since forgotten. Yet, it is not the Laws themselves that have the ability to alter our futures. Unless we consciously choose to use them, they cannot assist us in our healing process. It is the extent to which we are able to put these laws into practice that will allow us to increase the quality of our experiences, of our days and of our lives.

Final Summary

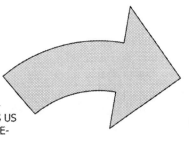

PRACTICING SELF-
ACCEPTANCE ALLOWS US
TO SHIFT FROM A DE-
SYNERGISTIC
RELATIONSHIP WITH
FOOD TO A SYNERGISTIC
RELATIONSHIP WITH
OURSELVES.
PHASE II

OPTIMIZING OUR
RELATIONSHIP WITH
FOOD (AND NOT
FOCUSING ON IT)
ALLOWS US TO DEAL
DIRECTLY WITH OUR
EMOTIONS.
PHASE I

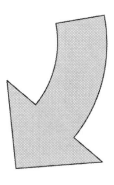

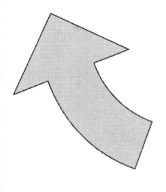

DEALING DIRECTLY WITH
OUR EMOTIONS MEANS
WE DON'T NEED TO USE
FOOD TO MODERATE
OUR FEELINGS.
PHASE III

Create Your Own Laws Of Gravity

I invite you to use these laws to assist you in creating your own synergistic path and I genuinely wish you the best of luck on your journey!

NEGATIVE CYCLE	POSITIVE CYCLE

ABOUT THE AUTHOR

Robin Ashley Long started off her career as a Chartered Accountant. In 1995, she returned to school to complete her Masters Degree in Counselling Psychology and to pursue a career that held greater meaning for her. She currently runs a private therapy practice in Toronto. She has worked with individuals who have struggled with dieting and body image concerns for over 15 years. Robin has provided both group and individual counselling, run support groups, published and lectured on the topic.

In addition to Robin's private practice, she works in the field of Industrial Psychology, where she assists Corporations in their Human Capital procurement, development and retention.

In 1992, Robin created, *The Great Escape,* a program that details the journey out of the "diet zone" for those struggling within the "diet chamber". Since then, she has used this program to work with hundreds of individuals who battle with weight, body image and eating issues. It is through her work with these individuals that certain "truisms" became readily apparent. Individuals appeared to follow certain forces of nature, regardless of where they were on the dieting spectrum. Anorexic and compulsive over-eaters alike, experience the same psychological patterns while exhibiting related, yet unique behaviours. *The Laws of Gravity* makes sense of these shared experiences.

To contact Robin Ashley Long directly:

www.Pro-ActiveCounselling.com

rlong@Pro-ActiveCounselling.com